AF350230

Table of Contents

Wellness on your plate

Conscious eating for a better life

Copyright ©

The content of this book, is protected by copyright laws and international treaties. All rights are reserved. No part of this publication may be reproduced, stored in a retrieval system, or transmitted in any form or by any means—electronic, mechanical, photocopying, recording, or otherwise—without the prior written permission of the copyright holders.

All efforts have been made to ensure the accuracy of the information presented in this book. However, the authors and the publisher do not assume responsibility for any errors or omissions.

James Thur – 2023 ©

Chapter 1: Understanding Conscious Eating

1.1 Introduction to Conscious Eating

In the hustle and bustle of modern life, we often find ourselves mindlessly munching on food while juggling multiple tasks. We eat on the go, distracted by screens, and rush through meals without even realizing what we're putting into our bodies. As a result, our relationship with food has become mechanical and devoid of true connection.

But what if we could change this? What if we could transform our eating habits into a mindful and conscious experience that nurtures not just our bodies but also our minds and souls? Welcome to the world of conscious eating, a profound approach to nourishing ourselves that goes beyond mere sustenance.

Conscious eating is about being present and aware of every aspect of the food we consume. It involves understanding where our food comes from, how it was grown or produced, and the impact it has on our bodies and the environment. This practice encourages us to savor every bite, to relish the flavors and textures, and to appreciate the nourishment that food provides.

One of the fundamental aspects of conscious eating is acknowledging the interconnection between what we eat and how we feel. Our bodies are intricate systems, and the food we consume serves as the fuel for our physical and mental well-being. When we eat with consciousness, we are better able to identify how different foods affect us, both positively and negatively.

Moreover, conscious eating is not about rigid diets or strict rules. It doesn't require us to label foods as "good" or "bad." Instead, it fosters a balanced approach that encourages us to listen to our bodies and respond to their unique needs. We learn to discern hunger from emotional triggers and to give ourselves permission to indulge in occasional treats without guilt.

To truly embrace conscious eating, we must also recognize the social and environmental implications of our food choices. It involves supporting local and sustainable food systems, reducing food waste, and appreciating the efforts of farmers and producers who bring nourishment to our plates.

In this journey towards conscious eating, we embark on a path of self-discovery. We become more attuned to our bodies and how different foods impact our energy levels, mood, and overall health. As we tune into our bodies, we develop a deeper sense of gratitude for the food we eat and the Earth that provides it.

Conscious eating is not an overnight transformation; it's a gradual shift in mindset and habits. It requires patience, self-compassion, and a willingness to explore new foods and culinary experiences. It's about celebrating food in all its diversity and richness while understanding its profound impact on our well-being.

Throughout this book, we will delve into the principles and practices of conscious eating. We will explore how to select wholesome foods that nourish us from the inside out, and we'll uncover the art of mindful eating, enabling us to savor each meal with joy and gratitude. We will also address the emotional aspects of eating and learn how to break free from unhealthy patterns that no longer serve us.

Beyond our personal transformation, conscious eating has the power to create a ripple effect of positive change in our communities and the world. By becoming more conscious of what we put on our plates, we can make choices that support sustainable practices and promote a healthier planet for future generations.

So, let us embark on this journey together, as we embrace the beauty of conscious eating and its profound impact on our well-being. As we develop a deeper connection with the food we eat, we open the door to a more fulfilling and balanced life, one delicious bite at a time. Let's savor this adventure and uncover the transformative power of wellness on our plates.

1.2 The Mind-Body Connection in Nutrition

In the fast-paced world we live in, it's easy to overlook the profound connection between what we eat and how we feel. However, the link between nutrition and our overall well-being goes far beyond mere physical sustenance. The food we consume plays a vital role in shaping our mental and emotional states, influencing everything from our mood and energy levels to our cognitive function and stress levels.

At the heart of this relationship lies the concept of the mind-body connection. The mind and body are intricately intertwined, and what we put into our bodies directly impacts our mental and emotional states. When we nourish ourselves with wholesome, nutrient-rich foods, we provide the essential building blocks for optimal brain function and emotional balance.

One of the key players in the mind-body connection is the gut-brain axis. The gut, often referred to as the "second brain," houses a complex network of neurons that communicate with our central nervous system. This connection between the gut and the brain is bidirectional, meaning that the state of our gut health can influence our mental well-being, and vice versa.

For instance, when we consume highly processed and sugary foods, it can lead to imbalances in our gut microbiome—the diverse community of microorganisms residing in our digestive tract. These imbalances can trigger inflammation and affect the production of neurotransmitters like serotonin, which plays a crucial role in regulating mood and emotions. As a result, poor dietary choices may contribute to feelings of anxiety, depression, and mood swings.

On the other hand, adopting a diet rich in whole foods, such as fruits, vegetables, whole grains, and healthy fats, supports a flourishing gut microbiome. This, in turn, can enhance the production of neurotransmitters that promote feelings of well-being, relaxation, and happiness. It's no wonder that many studies have highlighted the significant impact of the Mediterranean diet—an eating pattern abundant in fresh produce and healthy fats—on reducing the risk of depression and cognitive decline.

Moreover, the mind-body connection also influences how we perceive hunger and satiety. Emotional states can trigger overeating or loss of appetite, leading to unhealthy eating patterns. Stress, for example, can lead to emotional eating, where we seek comfort in food as a coping mechanism. Conversely, chronic stress can suppress appetite and disrupt our digestive processes, leading to nutrient malabsorption and related health issues.

By cultivating conscious eating habits, we can better understand and address these emotional triggers. Mindful eating practices help us recognize the difference between emotional hunger and physical hunger, allowing us to make more conscious choices about what and when to eat. Tuning into our bodies' signals enables us to nourish ourselves in a way that supports both our physical and emotional needs.

The mind-body connection in nutrition also extends to the realm of cognitive function and brain health. Certain nutrients, such as omega-3 fatty acids, antioxidants, and B vitamins, play crucial roles in supporting brain health and cognitive performance. These nutrients aid in neuroplasticity—the brain's ability to form new connections and adapt to changes.

Conversely, a diet high in trans fats, refined sugars, and processed foods can contribute to inflammation and oxidative stress in the brain, potentially impairing cognitive function and increasing the risk of neurodegenerative diseases.

Recognizing the impact of nutrition on cognitive health, researchers have explored the concept of "brain-boosting foods." Blueberries, for instance, are rich in antioxidants that may improve memory and cognitive function. Nuts and seeds provide essential fats and nutrients that support brain health. Dark leafy greens are abundant in vitamins and minerals that promote brain function and protect against cognitive decline.

In summary, the mind-body connection in nutrition is a profound and intricate relationship that significantly influences our overall well-being. By choosing to eat consciously and mindfully, we empower ourselves to nourish our bodies and minds in a way that supports optimal health and vitality. Taking the time to understand this connection and make informed choices about the foods we consume can lead us towards a more balanced, energized, and emotionally resilient life.

1.3 Benefits of Conscious Eating for Overall Wellness

Conscious eating is not just a passing dietary trend; it is a transformative lifestyle approach that can significantly impact our overall wellness. By becoming more aware and intentional about the food we put on our plates, we unlock a multitude of benefits that extend far beyond the physical aspect of nourishment.

Enhanced Nutritional Intake: When we practice conscious eating, we prioritize nutrient-dense foods that provide essential vitamins, minerals, and antioxidants. Filling our plates with colorful fruits and vegetables, whole grains, lean proteins, and healthy fats ensures that our bodies receive the necessary nutrients to function optimally.

Improved Digestion: Mindful eating involves savoring each bite and thoroughly chewing our food. This aids the digestive process by breaking down food more effectively and allowing our bodies to absorb nutrients more efficiently. Moreover, conscious eating encourages us to listen to our bodies' hunger and fullness cues, preventing overeating and reducing digestive discomfort.

Weight Management: Conscious eating is not about strict dieting but rather about attuning to our body's needs. By developing a deeper connection with our hunger and satiety signals, we can better regulate our food intake and maintain a healthy weight without resorting to restrictive measures.

Reduced Emotional Eating: Emotional eating often stems from an attempt to cope with stress, boredom, or other emotional triggers. Through conscious eating practices, we learn to recognize emotional hunger and find alternative ways to address our emotions without turning to food for comfort.

Heightened Mindfulness: As we become more mindful of our eating habits, we cultivate a heightened sense of awareness in other aspects of our lives. Mindfulness extends beyond the dinner table and spills over into our daily routines, enhancing our overall well-being.

Balanced Blood Sugar Levels: Conscious eating encourages us to choose whole, unprocessed foods, which help stabilize blood sugar levels and reduce the risk of developing insulin resistance and type 2 diabetes.

Increased Energy Levels: Nutrient-rich foods provide a steady source of energy, preventing energy spikes and crashes commonly associated with sugary and processed foods. With conscious eating, we experience sustained energy levels throughout the day.

Improved Mood and Mental Health: The gut-brain connection in conscious eating plays a pivotal role in supporting mental health. A diet rich in probiotics and fiber from plant-based foods can positively influence mood and reduce symptoms of anxiety and depression.

Enhanced Immune Function: A well-nourished body is better equipped to defend itself against infections and diseases.

Conscious eating strengthens the immune system, helping us stay healthy and ward off illnesses.

Connection to Nature: Embracing conscious eating encourages us to understand where our food comes from and the impact of our food choices on the environment. This fosters a deeper appreciation for nature and the interconnectedness of all living beings.

Sustainable Practices: Conscious eating aligns with sustainable and eco-friendly food choices. By supporting local farmers and opting for seasonal produce, we contribute to reducing our carbon footprint and preserving the planet for future generations.

Long-term Health Benefits: Adopting conscious eating as a way of life can lead to long-term health benefits, including a reduced risk of chronic diseases such as heart disease, certain cancers, and obesity.

Enhanced Self-Reflection: By paying attention to our eating habits, we gain insights into our relationship with food and our bodies. This self-reflection empowers us to make positive changes and cultivate a healthier mindset.

In conclusion, conscious eating offers a holistic approach to nutrition and overall wellness. By nourishing our bodies with intention, mindfulness, and gratitude, we unlock a myriad of physical, mental, and emotional benefits. Beyond the immediate impact on our health, conscious eating paves the way for a deeper connection with ourselves, our communities, and the planet we call home. It is a journey of self-discovery and transformation that enriches not only our plates but our lives as a whole.

13

Chapter 2: Nourishing Your Body with Wholesome Foods

2.1 Choosing Nutrient-Dense Foods

In the pursuit of conscious eating and overall wellness, one of the fundamental pillars is the selection of nutrient-dense foods. Nutrient density refers to the amount of essential nutrients—such as vitamins, minerals, protein, and healthy fats—found in a particular food relative to its calorie content. Opting for nutrient-dense foods ensures that we are fueling our bodies with vital nutrients without excess calories, promoting optimal health and vitality.

When we prioritize nutrient-dense foods, we nourish our bodies at a cellular level, providing the building blocks necessary for various biological processes. These foods not only support our physical health but also play a significant role in maintaining cognitive function, supporting immune function, and promoting healthy growth and development.

So, how do we identify and incorporate nutrient-dense foods into our diets?

Colorful Fruits and Vegetables: A rainbow of fruits and vegetables represents a diverse array of nutrients. Brightly colored produce, such as berries, leafy greens, sweet potatoes, and bell peppers, are rich in antioxidants, vitamins, and minerals. These powerful plant compounds protect our cells from damage and support overall well-being.

Whole Grains: Opt for whole grains over refined grains to maximize nutrient intake. Whole grains like quinoa, brown rice, oats, and whole wheat contain fiber, B vitamins, and essential minerals that contribute to better digestion and sustained energy levels.

Lean Proteins: Include lean sources of protein in your diet, such as poultry, fish, tofu, beans, and legumes. These options provide essential amino acids, promoting muscle health and repair, as well as contributing to satiety and blood sugar regulation.

Healthy Fats: Incorporate sources of healthy fats like avocados, nuts, seeds, and olive oil into your meals. These fats provide essential omega-3 fatty acids and contribute to heart health, brain function, and overall inflammation reduction.

Dairy and Dairy Alternatives: If you consume dairy, choose low-fat or unsweetened options like Greek yogurt or fortified plant-based alternatives. These choices provide calcium, vitamin D, and other nutrients crucial for bone health.

Nutrient-Dense Snacks: Snack smartly with nutrient-dense options like raw vegetables with hummus, a handful of nuts, or a piece of fruit. Avoid processed snacks with empty calories and limited nutritional value.

Hydration: Stay hydrated with water, herbal teas, and infused water. Proper hydration is vital for overall health and helps maintain optimal bodily functions.

Mindful Food Preparation: Be mindful of how you prepare your food. Cooking methods like steaming, roasting, and grilling preserve nutrients better than deep frying or excessive boiling.

Reading Food Labels: Take time to read food labels to identify the nutritional content and ingredients of packaged products. Look for items with minimal additives and artificial ingredients.

Variety and Balance: Embrace variety in your diet, consuming a diverse range of foods to ensure you obtain a wide spectrum of nutrients. Strive for balance, ensuring that each meal includes a combination of carbohydrates, proteins, healthy fats, and fiber.

While choosing nutrient-dense foods is crucial, it is essential to maintain a flexible and balanced approach to eating. Avoid rigid dieting rules or deprivation, as this can lead to an unhealthy relationship with food. Instead, focus on adding more nutrient-dense options to your meals, gradually crowding out less nutritious choices.

Conscious eating is not about perfection but about making thoughtful and informed decisions about the food we consume. By selecting nutrient-dense foods, we support our bodies in functioning optimally, boost our energy levels, and enhance our overall well-being. Remember that small, consistent steps towards conscious eating can lead to significant and sustainable improvements in your health and happiness.

2.2 The Power of Fresh Fruits and Vegetables

In the realm of nutrient-dense foods, fresh fruits and vegetables stand as vibrant and powerful ambassadors. These natural wonders of the plant kingdom are brimming with essential vitamins, minerals, antioxidants, and phytochemicals that contribute to our overall well-being. Incorporating a colorful array of fresh produce into our diets is a cornerstone of conscious eating, unlocking a host of health benefits and culinary delights.

Abundance of Essential Nutrients: Fresh fruits and vegetables are nutritional powerhouses, providing a wide range of essential nutrients that are crucial for our bodies to function optimally. They are rich sources of vitamins, such as vitamin C, vitamin A, vitamin K, and folate, all of which play pivotal roles in various bodily processes. Additionally, minerals like potassium, magnesium, and calcium are abundant in fresh produce, supporting heart health, bone health, and muscle function.

Antioxidant-Rich Allies: Antioxidants are potent compounds found in fresh fruits and vegetables that combat oxidative stress and protect our cells from damage caused by free radicals. Berries, leafy greens, tomatoes, and citrus fruits are just a few examples of antioxidant-rich foods. Regular consumption of these foods can contribute to reduced inflammation, improved skin health, and a lowered risk of chronic diseases.

Heart Health Champions: Many fresh fruits and vegetables, such as leafy greens, berries, and citrus fruits, support cardiovascular health. They contain dietary fiber, which helps to lower cholesterol levels and maintain healthy blood pressure. Moreover, certain plant compounds, like flavonoids and polyphenols, found in fruits and vegetables have been linked to a reduced risk of heart disease.

Digestive Superstars: Fresh fruits and vegetables are excellent sources of dietary fiber, which is essential for healthy digestion. Fiber promotes regular bowel movements, prevents constipation, and supports gut health by nourishing beneficial gut bacteria. A diet rich in fiber can also help with weight management and reduce the risk of developing certain digestive disorders.

Hydration and Vitality: Many fruits and vegetables have high water content, contributing to hydration and overall vitality. Staying well-hydrated supports numerous bodily functions, including temperature regulation, nutrient transportation, and toxin elimination. Consuming water-rich produce like cucumbers, watermelon, and oranges can help keep us hydrated throughout the day.

Weight Management: Fresh fruits and vegetables are naturally low in calories and high in fiber, making them excellent allies for weight management. Including these foods in our meals and snacks can promote feelings of fullness, reducing the likelihood of overeating and supporting weight loss or maintenance goals.

Immune System Boosters: The vitamins and antioxidants found in fresh produce, especially vitamin C and vitamin A, play vital roles in bolstering our immune systems. Regularly consuming fruits and vegetables helps to strengthen our immune response, making us more resilient to infections and illnesses.

Mental and Emotional Well-Being: The nutrient-rich profile of fresh fruits and vegetables can have positive effects on our mental and emotional health. Certain nutrients, such as folate, vitamin B6, and magnesium, are involved in neurotransmitter production and regulation, influencing mood and cognitive function.

Culinary Creativity: Embracing fresh fruits and vegetables opens the door to endless culinary possibilities. From refreshing fruit salads to hearty vegetable stir-fries and vibrant smoothies, there is no shortage of delicious ways to incorporate these natural gems into our daily meals.

Environmental Impact: Choosing fresh, locally grown produce can have a positive impact on the environment. Supporting local farmers reduces the carbon footprint associated with long-distance food transportation, and choosing seasonal produce promotes more sustainable agricultural practices.

In summary, fresh fruits and vegetables offer a multitude of health benefits that contribute to our overall well-being. They are a gift from nature, providing us with nourishment, flavor, and vitality. By celebrating the vibrant colors and flavors of fresh produce, we can embark on a culinary journey that delights our taste buds and nurtures our bodies from the inside out. As we cultivate a deeper appreciation for the power of fresh fruits and vegetables, we embrace a conscious eating approach that not only benefits our own health but also supports the health of the planet we call home.

2.3 Emphasizing Whole Grains and Plant-Based Proteins

In the quest for conscious eating and a balanced diet, whole grains and plant-based proteins take center stage as nutritional powerhouses. These two essential components form the foundation of many traditional diets and have been linked to numerous health benefits. By incorporating whole grains and plant-based proteins into our meals, we can enhance our overall well-being while supporting sustainable and environmentally friendly food choices.

Whole Grains:

Whole grains are grains that retain all three parts of the grain kernel—the bran, germ, and endosperm. This retention ensures that the grain maintains its nutritional integrity, providing a wealth of vitamins, minerals, dietary fiber, and phytonutrients. Emphasizing whole grains over refined grains brings a plethora of health benefits:

Heart Health: Whole grains, such as oats, barley, and brown rice, are rich in soluble fiber, which can help lower cholesterol levels and reduce the risk of heart disease. The fiber in whole grains also supports healthy blood pressure and improved cardiovascular health.

Stable Blood Sugar Levels: The fiber content in whole grains slows down the absorption of sugar in the bloodstream, promoting stable blood sugar levels. This can be especially beneficial for individuals with diabetes or those seeking to manage their blood sugar.

Digestive Health: Whole grains are an excellent source of insoluble fiber, which supports healthy digestion and helps prevent constipation. A diet rich in whole grains promotes a healthy gut environment and encourages regular bowel movements.

Weight Management: The fiber and complex carbohydrates in whole grains contribute to feelings of fullness and satiety, making them a valuable addition to a weight management plan.

Nutrient-Rich: Whole grains provide essential nutrients like B vitamins, iron, magnesium, and zinc, supporting energy production, immune function, and overall vitality.

Lower Risk of Chronic Diseases: Consuming whole grains has been associated with a reduced risk of chronic diseases such as type 2 diabetes, certain cancers, and obesity.

Plant-Based Proteins:

Plant-based proteins offer a wealth of nutrients and can be a valuable source of protein for individuals following vegetarian, vegan, or flexitarian diets. Including a variety of plant-based proteins in our meals offers numerous health advantages:

Heart Health: Plant-based proteins, like legumes, nuts, and seeds, are typically lower in saturated fat than animal-based proteins. A diet rich in plant-based proteins can support heart health and lower the risk of heart disease.

Fiber-Packed: Many plant-based proteins, such as lentils, chickpeas, and quinoa, are also excellent sources of dietary fiber. Fiber aids in digestion, promotes gut health, and supports weight management.

Essential Nutrients: Plant-based proteins supply essential nutrients such as iron, calcium, potassium, and various vitamins. These nutrients play crucial roles in bone health, muscle function, and overall body maintenance.

Environmentally Friendly: Producing plant-based proteins generally requires fewer natural resources and produces lower greenhouse gas emissions compared to animal-based proteins. Incorporating more plant-based proteins into our diets can have a positive impact on the environment.

Lower Cholesterol: Plant-based proteins, particularly legumes like beans and lentils, have been shown to help lower cholesterol levels, reducing the risk of heart disease.

Reduced Cancer Risk: A diet rich in plant-based proteins has been associated with a decreased risk of certain types of cancer, such as colorectal cancer.

By emphasizing whole grains and plant-based proteins in our meals, we not only enhance our personal well-being but also contribute to a more sustainable and eco-friendly food system. These nutrient-rich foods form the building blocks of a balanced and conscious eating approach, providing us with energy, vitality, and a host of health benefits.

Incorporating whole grains can be as simple as replacing refined grains with whole grain alternatives like brown rice, whole wheat pasta, and quinoa. Similarly, embracing plant-based proteins can involve experimenting with legumes, tofu, tempeh, nuts, and seeds in a variety of delicious and satisfying dishes.

As we prioritize whole grains and plant-based proteins in our diets, we discover a world of culinary possibilities that not only nourish our bodies but also celebrate the diversity and abundance of nature's bounty. By making these wholesome choices, we empower ourselves to thrive, while also contributing to a healthier planet for generations to come.

Chapter 3: Mindful Eating Practices

3.1 The Art of Mindful Eating

In a world filled with distractions and a fast-paced lifestyle, eating has become a mindless activity for many of us. We often consume meals on autopilot, rushing through our plates while preoccupied with work, smartphones, or other tasks. As a result, we miss out on the profound connection that food offers us—to nourish not only our bodies but also our minds and souls. Mindful eating is an ancient practice that invites us to slow down, savor every bite, and bring a profound awareness to the experience of eating.

At its core, mindful eating is about cultivating a deeper relationship with food. It encourages us to pay attention to our thoughts, feelings, and bodily sensations while we eat, allowing us to become more attuned to our hunger and fullness cues. By engaging all of our senses, we can fully appreciate the colors, textures, flavors, and aromas of the food on our plates.

Mindful eating is not about imposing strict rules or adhering to specific diets. Instead, it is a flexible and individualized approach that encourages us to listen to our bodies and respond to their unique needs. It invites us to release judgment and guilt around food choices, promoting a more compassionate and nurturing relationship with ourselves.

Here are some key principles of the art of mindful eating:

Presence: Mindful eating begins with being fully present during meals. Before diving into our plates, we take a moment to pause, breathe, and tune into the present moment. Letting go of distractions, we create a space of presence and awareness.

Savoring the Experience: Rather than rushing through meals, we savor each bite, taking our time to chew slowly and mindfully. As we engage all of our senses, we can fully appreciate the tastes, textures, and aromas of the food we eat.

Listening to Hunger and Fullness: Mindful eating encourages us to listen to our bodies and recognize when we are truly hungry and when we are comfortably full. This awareness allows us to eat in alignment with our body's needs, avoiding overeating or undereating.

Non-Judgmental Awareness: Mindful eating invites us to observe our thoughts and emotions around food without judgment. We release the idea of "good" or "bad" foods and instead embrace an attitude of curiosity and acceptance.

Emotional Eating: By being mindful of our emotions, we can distinguish between physical hunger and emotional hunger. Mindful eating helps us find alternative ways to address emotional needs without turning to food for comfort.

Gratitude and Connection: Expressing gratitude for the food we have and the efforts that went into its preparation deepens our connection to the nourishment it provides. Mindful eating reminds us of the interconnectedness of all beings and the Earth that sustains us.

Honoring the Body: Mindful eating encourages us to honor our bodies' signals and respect our individual dietary preferences and restrictions. It empowers us to make choices that support our health and well-being.

Mindful Meal Preparation: The art of mindful eating extends beyond the act of eating itself. It includes mindful meal preparation, where we engage with the process of cooking and appreciate the ingredients that go into our dishes.

Practicing mindful eating can have numerous benefits for our physical, emotional, and mental well-being:

Weight Management: By paying attention to hunger and fullness cues, we can better regulate our food intake and avoid overeating, supporting healthy weight management.

Digestive Health: Mindful eating promotes better digestion by encouraging us to chew our food thoroughly and eat in a relaxed state.

Stress Reduction: Engaging in mindful eating can help reduce stress and anxiety, as it creates a moment of stillness and focus during meals.

Improved Relationship with Food: Mindful eating fosters a more positive and balanced relationship with food, freeing us from guilt and allowing us to enjoy eating without restrictions.

Enhanced Gratitude: By being mindful of the food we eat, we develop a deeper sense of gratitude for the nourishment it provides and the abundance in our lives.

Cultivating the art of mindful eating takes practice and patience. It is not about achieving perfection but rather embracing the journey of self-awareness and connection with our bodies. By incorporating mindful eating into our daily lives, we can transform our relationship with food and experience the joy and fulfillment that come from being fully present during the simple act of nourishing ourselves.

3.2 Practicing Intuitive Eating

Intuitive eating is a revolutionary approach to nourishing our bodies that encourages us to tune inwards and trust our internal cues when it comes to food choices. It is a stark departure from traditional dieting and restrictive eating patterns, as it prioritizes listening to our bodies' natural hunger and fullness signals. The intuitive eating philosophy is founded on the belief that our bodies possess an inherent wisdom, guiding us towards the foods and quantities that best support our unique needs.

At the core of intuitive eating is the rejection of external rules and restrictions that often accompany traditional diets. Instead, it fosters a sense of autonomy and self-empowerment, encouraging individuals to make food choices based on what feels nourishing, satisfying, and enjoyable. Here are some key principles of practicing intuitive eating:

Honor Your Hunger: Intuitive eating begins with recognizing and honoring our hunger cues. We learn to differentiate between physical hunger, which manifests as a gnawing sensation in the stomach, and emotional hunger, which stems from feelings of boredom, stress, or sadness.

Eat Mindfully: Engaging in mindful eating practices, we become fully present during meals, savoring each bite and appreciating the flavors and textures of the food. Mindful eating helps us cultivate a deeper connection with our food and promotes a sense of gratitude for the nourishment it provides.

Respect Fullness: Intuitive eating empowers us to stop eating when we feel comfortably full, rather than finishing our plates out of habit or obligation. Respecting fullness cues prevents overeating and supports a more balanced relationship with food.

Embrace Food Neutrality: Intuitive eating encourages us to release judgment around food choices, embracing a neutral perspective. Foods are neither "good" nor "bad" but simply choices we make based on our preferences and needs at any given moment.

Reject Diet Culture: Practicing intuitive eating involves rejecting the harmful influences of diet culture, which perpetuates unrealistic beauty standards and promotes restrictive eating patterns. Instead, intuitive eating fosters body acceptance and the celebration of diverse body shapes and sizes.

Cope with Emotions without Food: Intuitive eating helps us find alternative ways to cope with emotions and stress, without turning to food for comfort. We learn to explore and address our emotions directly, nurturing ourselves in holistic ways that support emotional well-being.

Discover Satisfaction: Intuitive eating encourages us to seek pleasure and satisfaction in our meals. We explore different foods and flavors, allowing ourselves to indulge in occasional treats without guilt.

Trust Your Body: Perhaps the most crucial aspect of intuitive eating is developing trust in our bodies' wisdom. Instead of relying on external rules and guidelines, we turn inward and trust that our bodies know what they need to thrive.

The benefits of practicing intuitive eating extend far beyond improved relationships with food. This approach can have significant positive impacts on both physical and mental health:

Improved Self-Esteem: Embracing intuitive eating fosters self-acceptance and boosts self-esteem, as individuals no longer feel controlled by external dieting rules.

Healthier Metabolism: By eating in response to genuine hunger and fullness signals, our metabolism can regulate more efficiently, promoting better energy balance.

Balanced Weight: Intuitive eating encourages weight stabilization, as it helps individuals find their natural, healthy weight without engaging in restrictive dieting.

Enhanced Mental Health: Letting go of dieting and body image obsessions can lead to reduced anxiety, depression, and disordered eating patterns.

Body Trust and Intuition: Practicing intuitive eating strengthens our connection with our bodies, helping us better understand and respond to their needs.

Sustainable Approach: Intuitive eating is a lifelong approach to eating that can be sustained throughout various life stages and circumstances.

Practicing intuitive eating is a journey that requires patience, self-compassion, and a willingness to challenge societal norms around food and body image. It involves unlearning harmful dieting behaviors and embracing a more intuitive and compassionate way of nourishing ourselves. By honoring our bodies' innate wisdom and adopting a mindful, non-judgmental approach to eating, we can cultivate a healthier and more fulfilling relationship with food and, ultimately, with ourselves.

3.3 Mindful Eating for Weight Management and Digestion

Mindful eating is not only a transformative approach to our relationship with food but also a powerful tool for weight management and improved digestion. By practicing mindful eating, we can develop a more conscious and balanced approach to nourishing our bodies, leading to healthier eating habits and a greater sense of well-being.

Weight Management:

Mindful eating offers a sustainable and effective approach to weight management without the need for restrictive diets or calorie counting. By paying attention to our body's hunger and fullness signals, we can prevent overeating and emotional eating, both of which can contribute to weight gain.

In mindful eating, we learn to distinguish between true physical hunger and emotional hunger. Emotional eating often arises from stress, boredom, or other emotions, leading us to seek comfort in food. By addressing emotional needs directly and finding alternative coping mechanisms, we can avoid using food as an emotional crutch.

Mindful eating also encourages us to savor our meals and be fully present during eating, allowing us to experience greater satisfaction with smaller portions. When we eat slowly and mindfully, we give our bodies time to signal when we are comfortably full, preventing overeating and promoting a healthier energy balance.

Moreover, by embracing food neutrality and releasing the guilt associated with certain foods, we reduce the likelihood of engaging in binge eating or cycles of deprivation and overindulgence. This balanced approach to eating supports a more stable and sustainable weight.

Improved Digestion:

Digestive health is closely linked to mindful eating practices. When we eat mindfully, we chew our food thoroughly, breaking it down into smaller pieces that are easier for the digestive system to process. Properly chewing our food supports the release of digestive enzymes, facilitating nutrient absorption and reducing the risk of indigestion and bloating.

Mindful eating also encourages us to eat in a relaxed state, free from stress and distractions. Stress can negatively impact digestion, leading to issues like irritable bowel syndrome (IBS) and other digestive disorders. By creating a calm and mindful eating environment, we support optimal digestion and nutrient assimilation.

Additionally, mindful eating helps us identify and address food sensitivities or intolerances. By paying attention to how our bodies respond to different foods, we can better understand which ones may cause digestive discomfort or inflammation.

Furthermore, by incorporating more plant-based foods and whole grains into our meals, as encouraged by mindful eating, we promote better digestion. These fiber-rich foods support healthy gut bacteria, prevent constipation, and aid in waste elimination.

Overall, the mindfulness and intentionality of mindful eating contribute to improved digestion and reduced digestive discomfort.

In conclusion, mindful eating offers valuable tools for weight management and improved digestion. By practicing conscious awareness of our body's hunger and fullness signals, we can support a healthy weight without resorting to restrictive diets. Embracing food neutrality and letting go of guilt around eating enables us to cultivate a more balanced and sustainable approach to nourishing our bodies.

Moreover, mindful eating fosters better digestion by promoting proper chewing, a relaxed eating environment, and a focus on whole, nutrient-rich foods. By nourishing our bodies with intention and awareness, we can unlock the transformative power of mindful eating, leading to improved well-being and a deeper connection with ourselves and the food we eat.

Chapter 4: Cultivating a Balanced Relationship with Food

4.1 Overcoming Emotional Eating

Emotional eating is a common phenomenon in today's fast-paced and stress-filled world. It involves using food as a way to cope with emotions such as stress, anxiety, sadness, boredom, or even happiness. When faced with challenging emotions, turning to food for comfort can provide temporary relief, but it often leads to feelings of guilt, regret, and a cycle of emotional eating.

Identifying and overcoming emotional eating is crucial for fostering a healthier relationship with food and supporting overall well-being. Here are some strategies to help overcome emotional eating:

Mindful Awareness: The first step in overcoming emotional eating is to become more mindful and aware of our eating habits. Pay attention to when and why you reach for food. Are you truly hungry, or is it driven by emotions? Keeping a food journal can be helpful in recognizing patterns and triggers.

Identify Emotional Triggers: Emotional eating often follows specific triggers or events. Stressful days at work, relationship issues, or feelings of loneliness can lead to reaching for comfort foods. By identifying these triggers, we can find healthier ways to cope with emotions.

Find Alternative Coping Mechanisms: Rather than turning to food, seek alternative ways to cope with emotions. Engage in activities that bring joy and relaxation, such as taking a walk, practicing yoga, reading, or spending time with loved ones.

Emotional Check-Ins: Before reaching for food, pause and check in with yourself. Ask if you are physically hungry or if you are seeking food to fill an emotional void. By creating a moment of awareness, you can make more conscious choices about eating.

Develop Healthy Habits: Cultivate a routine of self-care and stress management that doesn't involve food. Regular exercise, sufficient sleep, and relaxation techniques can all contribute to a more balanced emotional state.

Practice Mindful Eating: Incorporate mindful eating practices into your meals. Slow down and savor the flavors, textures, and aromas of your food. By eating mindfully, you can find pleasure and satisfaction in smaller portions, reducing the likelihood of overeating.

Seek Support: Overcoming emotional eating may require support from friends, family, or professionals. Consider talking to a therapist or counselor who can help you address emotional triggers and develop healthier coping strategies.

Create a Supportive Environment: Surround yourself with an environment that encourages mindful eating and healthy choices. Stock your kitchen with nutritious foods, and remove or limit access to trigger foods.

Practice Self-Compassion: Be kind to yourself throughout the process of overcoming emotional eating. Avoid self-criticism or harsh judgment. Embrace the journey of growth and self-discovery with compassion and understanding.

Be Patient: Changing ingrained habits takes time and effort. Be patient with yourself as you work on overcoming emotional eating. Celebrate small victories and view setbacks as opportunities for learning and growth.

It's important to remember that occasional emotional eating is normal and part of being human. The goal is not to eliminate emotional eating entirely but to develop a healthier balance and find alternative ways to cope with emotions. By adopting mindful eating practices and addressing emotional triggers, we can break free from the cycle of emotional eating and build a more nourishing and sustainable relationship with food.

Overcoming emotional eating is a journey of self-awareness and self-compassion. By learning to recognize and address emotional triggers, finding healthier coping mechanisms, and embracing mindful eating practices, we can foster a more balanced and fulfilling approach to nourishing our bodies and minds. With patience, support, and self-love, we can conquer emotional eating and create a more harmonious and joyful relationship with food.

4.2 Redefining Treats and Indulgences

In the realm of conscious eating, the notion of treats and indulgences takes on a new and empowered meaning. Traditionally, treats have been associated with foods that are considered "unhealthy" or "off-limits," leading to feelings of guilt and shame when indulging in them. However, redefining treats and indulgences is about embracing a balanced and compassionate approach to enjoying food while honoring our bodies' needs and preferences.

Letting Go of Food Guilt: Redefining treats involves letting go of the guilt and negative associations often attached to certain foods. Instead of labeling foods as "good" or "bad," we adopt a more neutral perspective, recognizing that all foods can be enjoyed in moderation.

Intentional Indulgences: Rather than mindlessly indulging in treats, we embrace the concept of intentional indulgences. This means consciously choosing treats that genuinely bring joy and pleasure, without feeling guilty about enjoying them.

Mindful Enjoyment: When we redefine treats, we practice mindful enjoyment. We savor each bite, fully immersing ourselves in the flavors and textures of the treat. By eating mindfully, we enhance the experience and avoid overeating out of mindless habit.

Balanced Choices: Redefining treats involves finding a balance between nourishing our bodies with nutrient-dense foods and allowing ourselves occasional indulgences. Moderation is key, as enjoying treats in the context of an overall healthy diet can be a sustainable and guilt-free approach.

Avoiding Restrictive Mindsets: Restrictive eating patterns can lead to feelings of deprivation and unhealthy relationships with food. Redefining treats means breaking free from rigid rules and embracing a more flexible and intuitive approach to eating.

Embracing Occasional Indulgences: It's important to recognize that indulging in treats occasionally is a normal and enjoyable part of life. Occasional indulgences can be a source of pleasure and connection, allowing us to celebrate special occasions and enjoy social gatherings.

Nourishing the Soul: Redefining treats acknowledges that food can nourish not only our bodies but also our souls. Treats can be a source of comfort, celebration, and cultural connection, adding richness and joy to our lives.

Food as Celebration: We redefine treats as a form of celebration rather than a means of escape or emotional comfort. Treating ourselves to a favorite dessert or special meal can be a way to acknowledge accomplishments or create cherished memories with loved ones.

Self-Compassion: Redefining treats involves practicing self-compassion and self-kindness. If we occasionally indulge in foods that may not be as nutrient-dense, we avoid self-criticism and guilt. Instead, we focus on enjoying the experience and nurturing our well-being in all aspects of life.

Moderation and Balance: Above all, redefining treats is about finding balance and moderation in our eating habits. By incorporating nutrient-dense foods as the foundation of our diet and allowing space for occasional treats, we create a sustainable and enjoyable way of nourishing ourselves.

As we redefine treats and indulgences, we embrace a healthier and more positive relationship with food. It is not about completely avoiding certain foods but about shifting our mindset and making conscious choices that align with our well-being and values. By embracing mindful enjoyment, letting go of guilt, and finding balance in our eating habits, we can celebrate the joy of eating and create a more nourishing and pleasurable relationship with food. Redefining treats is a journey of self-discovery and self-compassion, allowing us to fully embrace the beauty and abundance of food in all its forms.

4.3 Breaking Free from Restrictive Dieting Mentality

The restrictive dieting mentality has long been ingrained in our culture as a means to achieve a certain body shape or weight. It often involves following rigid and unsustainable eating patterns that promise quick results but can lead to a host of physical and emotional consequences. Breaking free from the restrictive dieting mentality is essential for cultivating a healthy relationship with food, supporting overall well-being, and nurturing a positive body image.

Embracing Individuality: One of the first steps in breaking free from restrictive dieting mentality is embracing our unique individuality. Each person has a different body composition, metabolism, and nutritional needs. Instead of comparing ourselves to others, we learn to honor and respect our bodies for their inherent wisdom and beauty.

Rejecting Quick Fixes: Restrictive diets often promise quick fixes and rapid weight loss. However, these drastic changes can be detrimental to our health and lead to yo-yo dieting. Breaking free from this mentality involves understanding that sustainable and lasting changes take time and patience.

Fostering a Healthy Mindset: Breaking free from restrictive dieting involves shifting our mindset from a focus on weight and appearance to prioritizing health and well-being. We recognize that health is not solely determined by the number on the scale but by nourishing our bodies with nutrient-dense foods and engaging in regular physical activity.

Listening to Our Bodies: Restrictive dieting often teaches us to ignore our body's hunger and fullness cues and instead rely on external rules and guidelines. Breaking free from this mentality means relearning how to listen to our bodies and respond to their unique needs. This includes eating when we are hungry, stopping when we are satisfied, and being attuned to our body's signals of fatigue, hunger, and fullness.

Cultivating Intuitive Eating: Intuitive eating is a powerful tool for breaking free from restrictive dieting. It involves tuning into our body's natural hunger and fullness cues, eating mindfully, and making food choices based on what feels nourishing and satisfying. Intuitive eating empowers us to trust our bodies and build a positive and balanced relationship with food.

Honoring Food Preferences: Restrictive dieting often demonizes certain foods and promotes an all-or-nothing approach. Breaking free from this mentality means honoring our food preferences and allowing ourselves to enjoy a wide variety of foods, including treats and indulgences, without guilt or shame.

Nurturing Body Positivity: Breaking free from restrictive dieting means embracing body positivity and challenging unrealistic beauty standards. We celebrate our bodies for their strength, resilience, and unique beauty, regardless of their size or shape.

Building a Supportive Environment: Surrounding ourselves with a supportive and positive environment is crucial for breaking free from restrictive dieting. This may include seeking the support of friends, family, or a professional counselor who can help us challenge harmful beliefs and develop a healthier mindset.

Self-Compassion and Forgiveness: As we break free from restrictive dieting, we may encounter setbacks and challenges. Practicing self-compassion and forgiveness allows us to approach these moments with kindness and understanding, rather than self-criticism.

Embracing a Holistic Approach: Breaking free from restrictive dieting involves embracing a holistic approach to health and well-being. This includes nourishing not only our bodies but also our minds and souls through self-care practices, stress management, and finding joy in various aspects of life.

Breaking free from restrictive dieting mentality is a transformative journey that empowers us to reclaim our relationship with food and our bodies. By embracing individuality, fostering a healthy mindset, and cultivating intuitive eating practices, we can nurture a positive body image and support our overall well-being. As we let go of restrictive rules and embrace a more compassionate and balanced approach to nourishment, we discover the freedom and joy of living a life that is truly in harmony with our bodies and souls.

Chapter 5: Sustainable Eating for Personal and Planetary Health

5.1 Choosing Locally Sourced and Seasonal Foods

In the pursuit of conscious eating, the choices we make about the foods we consume have far-reaching impacts beyond our own well-being. Opting for locally sourced and seasonal foods is not only beneficial for our health but also for the environment, local economies, and our connection to the natural world. Embracing this approach to food selection allows us to align our eating habits with sustainable practices, supporting a healthier planet and fostering a deeper appreciation for the food on our plates.

Environmental Benefits:

Choosing locally sourced and seasonal foods significantly reduces the carbon footprint associated with our meals. When food is sourced from nearby farms and producers, it requires less transportation and refrigeration, leading to lower greenhouse gas emissions. In contrast, food that is imported from distant locations often requires long-distance shipping and storage, contributing to pollution and climate change.

Seasonal eating is also more sustainable as it relies on natural growing cycles and minimizes the need for energy-intensive methods of production. By consuming foods that naturally thrive during specific seasons, we encourage a more balanced and environmentally friendly food system.

Supporting Local Communities:

Opting for locally sourced foods supports local farmers, growers, and artisans. Purchasing from nearby producers strengthens local economies, creating jobs and promoting sustainable agricultural practices. By investing in local food systems, we contribute to the resilience and vitality of our communities.

Fresher and Nutrient-Rich Foods:

Locally sourced foods are often fresher than those that travel long distances to reach us. Fruits and vegetables that are harvested closer to their ripening and consumption dates retain more nutrients, making them more nutritious and flavorful.

Seasonal eating also encourages a diverse and well-rounded diet. Consuming foods that are in season exposes us to a wide variety of nutrients and flavors throughout the year. As nature provides different produce during different seasons, we can enjoy a colorful and nutritious array of foods.

Connection to Nature:

Choosing locally sourced and seasonal foods deepens our connection to the natural world and the cycles of life. It reminds us of the rhythms of the earth and the interdependence between humans and the environment. By aligning our eating habits with nature's cycles, we cultivate a sense of gratitude for the abundance that the earth provides.

Preservation of Biodiversity:

Embracing seasonal eating contributes to the preservation of biodiversity. When we consume a diverse range of fruits and vegetables throughout the year, we support the cultivation of various plant species. This, in turn, helps protect agricultural biodiversity and ensures that traditional and heirloom varieties are not lost.

Adaptability and Creativity in the Kitchen:

Seasonal eating encourages adaptability and creativity in the kitchen. As we work with the produce available in each season, we discover new flavors, experiment with different recipes, and learn to appreciate the unique qualities of each ingredient.

Community Involvement:

Choosing locally sourced foods often opens the door to community-supported agriculture (CSA) and farmers' markets. Engaging with these local initiatives allows us to interact directly with the people who grow our food, fostering a sense of community and transparency in the food system.

Mindful Consumerism:

Opting for locally sourced and seasonal foods aligns with the principles of mindful consumerism. By consciously considering the origins and impact of the foods we purchase, we make choices that reflect our values and support sustainable and ethical practices.

Incorporating locally sourced and seasonal foods into our diets may require some adjustments, especially if we are used to having access to a wide range of foods year-round. However, the benefits, both for our well-being and the environment, make the transition well worth it. By choosing to embrace the rich offerings of each season and supporting local producers, we not only nourish our bodies but also become stewards of a more sustainable and resilient food system. Conscious eating, with an emphasis on locally sourced and seasonal foods, empowers us to make a positive impact on our health, communities, and the planet we call home.

5.2 Understanding the Impact of Food Choices on the Environment

Our food choices have a profound impact on the environment, far beyond what we may realize. As conscious eaters, it is essential to understand how our decisions about what we eat can either contribute to environmental degradation or support sustainable practices that promote a healthier planet.

Greenhouse Gas Emissions:

The food industry is a significant contributor to greenhouse gas emissions. Agriculture, livestock production, food processing, and transportation all play a role in emitting carbon dioxide, methane, and nitrous oxide, which trap heat in the atmosphere and contribute to global warming and climate change.

Animal agriculture, particularly intensive livestock farming, is a major source of methane, a potent greenhouse gas. Choosing plant-based meals and reducing our meat consumption can significantly lower our carbon footprint.

Land Use and Deforestation:

The demand for food, especially meat and animal feed, has led to extensive deforestation in many regions. Forests are cleared to create space for livestock grazing and crop cultivation, resulting in the loss of biodiversity and natural habitats for wildlife.

By supporting sustainably produced foods and reducing our meat consumption, we can help reduce the demand for agricultural expansion, thus mitigating the impact of deforestation on the environment.

Water Consumption:

The food industry is a major consumer of water resources. Agriculture, in particular, uses vast amounts of water for irrigation, which can deplete water sources and lead to water scarcity in regions with already limited access to water.

Opting for plant-based diets and choosing foods that are locally sourced can help reduce our water footprint. Fruits and vegetables generally require less water to produce compared to animal-based products.

Pollution and Chemical Use:

Conventional farming practices often rely on the heavy use of chemical fertilizers, pesticides, and herbicides. These chemicals can leach into the soil and waterways, causing pollution and harming ecosystems.

Supporting organic and regenerative farming practices can help minimize chemical use and promote healthier soils and ecosystems.

Food Waste:

Food waste is a significant environmental issue. When we waste food, we also waste the resources, energy, and water used to produce, process, and transport that food.

Reducing food waste at the consumer level can have a positive impact on the environment. Being mindful of portion sizes, planning meals, and using leftovers creatively are some ways to minimize food waste.

Plastic Packaging:

Packaging is a major source of plastic waste, which contributes to pollution and harm to marine life. Processed and convenience foods often come in single-use plastic packaging, which has a detrimental effect on the environment.

Choosing fresh, unpackaged foods and supporting businesses that prioritize sustainable packaging can help reduce plastic waste.

Loss of Biodiversity:

Industrial agriculture practices often focus on a limited number of high-yield crops, leading to a loss of biodiversity. This reduction in plant and animal diversity can negatively impact ecosystems and make food systems more vulnerable to disease and climate change.

Supporting diverse and locally adapted food varieties can help preserve biodiversity and support more resilient food systems.

Sustainable Seafood:

The seafood industry faces numerous challenges, including overfishing, bycatch (the unintended capture of non-target species), and habitat destruction. Choosing sustainably sourced seafood can help protect marine ecosystems and promote responsible fishing practices.

Understanding the environmental impact of our food choices empowers us to make more informed and sustainable decisions. By opting for plant-based meals, choosing locally sourced and seasonal foods, reducing food waste, and supporting sustainable farming and fishing practices, we can play an active role in promoting a more environmentally friendly and resilient food system. As conscious eaters, we have the power to contribute positively to the health of our planet and protect the precious resources that sustain us all.

5.3 Reducing Food Waste and Promoting Sustainable Practices

Food waste is a significant global issue that not only affects food security but also has a significant environmental impact. As conscious eaters, we have a crucial role in reducing food waste and promoting sustainable practices throughout the food supply chain.

Mindful Meal Planning:

One of the most effective ways to reduce food waste is through mindful meal planning. By planning our meals ahead of time, we can make a shopping list with the exact ingredients we need, avoiding impulse purchases and excess food that might go to waste.

Proper Storage and Preservation:

Properly storing and preserving food can extend its shelf life and reduce spoilage. Understanding the optimal storage conditions for different foods can help prevent them from going bad too quickly.

Using Leftovers Creatively:

Leftovers can be transformed into delicious new meals, reducing food waste and saving money. Get creative in the kitchen by turning last night's dinner into a new dish or incorporating leftovers into a salad or wrap.

Composting:

Composting is an eco-friendly way to dispose of food scraps and other organic waste. By composting, we divert food waste from landfills, where it would generate harmful greenhouse gases, and instead create nutrient-rich soil for gardening and agriculture.

Supporting Local Food Recovery Initiatives:

Many communities have food recovery initiatives that collect surplus food from restaurants, grocery stores, and other sources to distribute to those in need. Supporting and volunteering for these initiatives helps prevent perfectly good food from being wasted while assisting those facing food insecurity.

Sustainable Food Shopping:

When grocery shopping, we can make sustainable choices by opting for products with minimal packaging or choosing products in bulk. Additionally, supporting businesses that prioritize sustainable and environmentally friendly practices encourages more sustainable food production.

Reducing Excess Portions:

Restaurants and eateries often serve large portions, which can lead to food waste when diners can't finish their meals. By choosing smaller portions or sharing dishes, we can reduce food waste while supporting businesses that practice sustainable portioning.

Awareness of Expiration Dates:

Understanding expiration dates and "best before" labels can help us use up food before it goes bad. Many products are still safe to eat after their expiration dates, so learning to discern between spoilage and safe consumption is essential in reducing food waste.

Donating Excess Food:

When we find ourselves with excess food that we can't use or preserve, donating it to food banks or shelters is a meaningful way to prevent waste and support those in need.

Advocating for Sustainable Policies:

As conscious eaters, we can also advocate for sustainable food policies at the local, national, and global levels. Supporting initiatives that promote food waste reduction, sustainable farming practices, and responsible food distribution can drive positive change in the food system.

By adopting these practices and promoting sustainability, we can make a significant impact on reducing food waste and supporting a more resilient and sustainable food system. As conscious eaters, we have the power to influence the entire food supply chain, from production to consumption, and contribute to a more environmentally friendly and equitable world. Reducing food waste and promoting sustainable practices not only benefits us as individuals but also helps to protect the planet and ensure a more abundant and sustainable future for generations to come.

Conclusion: Embracing Conscious Eating for a Lifetime of Wellness

Conscious eating is not just a fleeting trend; it is a transformative and lifelong journey that nourishes not only our bodies but also our minds and souls. Throughout this exploration, we have delved into the various aspects of conscious eating, including understanding the impact of our food choices, cultivating a mindful and intuitive approach to eating, and embracing sustainable practices that support both our well-being and the health of the planet.

At the heart of conscious eating is the recognition that food is not merely fuel for our bodies but a source of connection, culture, and joy. It is about celebrating the abundance of nature and fostering a deep appreciation for the nourishment it provides. Conscious eating is an invitation to slow down, savor each bite, and be fully present during meals, allowing us to experience the full pleasure and satisfaction that food can bring.

By choosing nutrient-dense foods, embracing whole and unprocessed ingredients, and prioritizing locally sourced and seasonal produce, we align our food choices with the rhythms of nature. We become more attuned to the cycles of life and develop a profound connection to the earth that sustains us.

Intuitive eating, another pillar of conscious eating, empowers us to listen to our bodies' innate wisdom. By tuning into our hunger and fullness cues and recognizing the impact of emotions on our eating habits, we free ourselves from the constraints of restrictive dieting and create a healthier and more sustainable approach to nourishing our bodies.

Conscious eating also extends beyond the individual to encompass the global community. It is about understanding the environmental impact of our food choices and advocating for sustainable practices that protect the planet for future generations. By reducing food waste, supporting local farmers and producers, and promoting responsible food sourcing, we actively contribute to building a more resilient and equitable food system.

Throughout our conscious eating journey, we may encounter challenges and setbacks. It's essential to approach these moments with self-compassion, embracing the idea that mindful eating is not about perfection but progress. Every small step we take toward conscious eating makes a difference, both in our lives and in the world around us.

As we embark on this lifelong journey of conscious eating, let us remember that it is not a rigid set of rules but a flexible and adaptable approach to nourishment. It is about finding balance, joy, and a deeper connection to ourselves, each other, and the earth. It is about celebrating the diversity of food and culture, and the shared experience of sharing meals with loved ones.

In conclusion, embracing conscious eating is an invitation to reclaim our relationship with food, our bodies, and the natural world. It is a call to action to become stewards of our health and the health of the planet. By choosing to nourish ourselves mindfully and sustainably, we can create a lifetime of wellness, one meal at a time. Let us embark on this journey together, with curiosity, openness, and the knowledge that our choices, however small, have the power to shape a better and more compassionate world.